Everything You Need to Know About Anxiety Disorders

Causes ◆ Symptoms ◆ Treatment

Watch a video version:

https://www.youtube.com/watch?v=_UqiU1zNcig

This book is based on information and recommendations by the Department of Health, United States government.

Created By The Bizmove Health Team

Disclaimer

All the content found in this book was created for informational purposes only. The Content is not intended to be a substitute for professional medical advice, diagnosis, or treatment. Always seek the advice of your physician or other qualified health provider with any questions you may have regarding a medical condition. Never disregard professional medical advice or delay in seeking it because of something you have read in this book.

ISBN: 9798746884541

Everything You Need to Know About Anxiety Disorders

Occasional anxiety is an expected part of life. You might feel anxious when faced with a problem at work, before taking a test, or before making an important decision. But anxiety disorders involve more than temporary worry or fear. For a person with an anxiety disorder, the anxiety does not go away and can get worse over time. The symptoms can interfere with daily activities such as job performance, school work, and relationships.

There are several types of anxiety disorders, including generalized anxiety disorder, panic disorder, and various phobia-related disorders.

Signs and Symptoms

Generalized Anxiety Disorder

People with generalized anxiety disorder (GAD) display excessive anxiety or worry, most days for at least 6 months, about a number of things such as personal health, work, social interactions, and everyday routine life circumstances. The fear and anxiety can cause significant problems in areas of their life, such as social interactions, school, and work.

Generalized anxiety disorder symptoms include:

- Feeling restless, wound-up, or on-edge
- Being easily fatigued
- Having difficulty concentrating; mind going blank
- Being irritable
- Having muscle tension
- Difficulty controlling feelings of worry
- Having sleep problems, such as difficulty falling or staying asleep, restlessness, or unsatisfying sleep

Panic Disorder

People with panic disorder have recurrent unexpected panic attacks. Panic attacks are sudden periods of intense fear that come on quickly and reach their peak within minutes. Attacks can occur unexpectedly or can be brought on by a trigger, such as a feared object or situation.

During a panic attack, people may experience:

- Heart palpitations, a pounding heartbeat, or an accelerated heartrate
- Sweating
- Trembling or shaking

- Sensations of shortness of breath, smothering, or choking
- Feelings of impending doom
- Feelings of being out of control

People with panic disorder often worry about when the next attack will happen and actively try to prevent future attacks by avoiding places, situations, or behaviors they associate with panic attacks. Worry about panic attacks, and the effort spent trying to avoid attacks, cause significant problems in various areas of the person's life, including the development of agoraphobia (see below).

Phobia-related disorders

A *phobia* is an intense fear of—or aversion to—specific objects or situations. Although it can be realistic to be anxious in some circumstances, the fear people with phobias feel is out of proportion to the actual danger caused by the situation or object.

People with a phobia:

- May have an irrational or excessive worry about encountering the feared object or situation
- Take active steps to avoid the feared object or situation
- Experience immediate intense anxiety upon encountering the feared object or situation

- Endure unavoidable objects and situations with intense anxiety

There are several types of phobias and phobia-related disorders:

Specific Phobias (sometimes called simple phobias): As the name suggests, people who have a specific phobia have an intense fear of, or feel intense anxiety about, specific types of objects or situations. Some examples of specific phobias include the fear of:

- Flying
- Heights
- Specific animals, such as spiders, dogs, or snakes
- Receiving injections
- Blood

Social anxiety disorder (previously called social phobia): People with social anxiety disorder have a general intense fear of, or anxiety toward, social or performance situations. They worry that actions or behaviors associated with their anxiety will be negatively evaluated by others, leading them to feel embarrassed. This worry often causes people with social anxiety to avoid social situations. Social anxiety disorder can manifest in a range of situations, such as within the workplace or the school environment.

Agoraphobia: People with agoraphobia have an intense fear of two or more of the following situations:

- Using public transportation
- Being in open spaces
- Being in enclosed spaces
- Standing in line or being in a crowd
- Being outside of the home alone

People with agoraphobia often avoid these situations, in part, because they think being able to leave might be difficult or impossible in the event they have panic-like reactions or other embarrassing symptoms. In the most severe form of agoraphobia, an individual can become housebound.

Separation anxiety disorder: Separation anxiety is often thought of as something that only children deal with; however, adults can also be diagnosed with separation anxiety disorder. People who have separation anxiety disorder have fears about being parted from people to whom they are attached. They often worry that some sort of harm or something untoward will happen to their attachment figures while they are separated. This fear leads them to avoid being separated from their attachment figures and to avoid being alone. People with separation anxiety may have nightmares about being separated from attachment figures or experience physical symptoms when separation occurs or is anticipated.

Selective mutism: A somewhat rare disorder associated with anxiety is *selective mutism*. Selective mutism occurs when people fail to speak in specific social situations despite having normal language skills. Selective mutism usually occurs before the age of 5 and is often associated with extreme shyness, fear of social embarrassment, compulsive traits, withdrawal, clinging behavior, and temper tantrums. People diagnosed with selective mutism are often also diagnosed with other anxiety disorders.

Risk Factors

Researchers are finding that both genetic and environmental factors contribute to the risk of developing an anxiety disorder. Although the risk factors for each type of anxiety disorder can vary, some general risk factors for all types of anxiety disorders include:

- Temperamental traits of shyness or behavioral inhibition in childhood
- Exposure to stressful and negative life or environmental events in early childhood or adulthood

- A history of anxiety or other mental illnesses in biological relatives
- Some physical health conditions, such as thyroid problems or heart arrhythmias, or caffeine or other substances/medications, can produce or aggravate anxiety symptoms; a physical health examination is helpful in the evaluation of a possible anxiety disorder.

Treatments and Therapies

Anxiety disorders are generally treated with psychotherapy, medication, or both. There are many ways to treat anxiety and people should work with their doctor to choose the treatment that is best for them.

Psychotherapy

Psychotherapy or "talk therapy" can help people with anxiety disorders. To be effective, psychotherapy must be directed at the person's specific anxieties and tailored to his or her needs.

Cognitive Behavioral Therapy

Cognitive Behavioral Therapy (CBT) is an example of one type of psychotherapy that can help people with anxiety disorders. It teaches people different ways of thinking, behaving, and reacting to anxiety-producing and fearful objects and situations. CBT can also help people learn and practice social skills, which is vital for treating social anxiety disorder.

Cognitive therapy and exposure therapy are two CBT methods that are often used, together or by themselves, to treat social anxiety disorder. Cognitive therapy focuses on identifying, challenging, and then neutralizing unhelpful or distorted thoughts underlying anxiety disorders. Exposure therapy focuses on confronting the fears underlying an anxiety disorder to help people engage in activities they have been avoiding. Exposure therapy is sometimes used along with relaxation exercises and/or imagery.

CBT can be conducted individually or with a group of people who have similar difficulties. Often "homework" is assigned for participants to complete between sessions.

Medication

Medication does not cure anxiety disorders but can help relieve symptoms. Medication for anxiety is prescribed by doctors, such as a psychiatrist or primary care provider. Some states also allow psychologists who have received specialized training to prescribe psychiatric medications. The most common classes of medications used to combat anxiety disorders are anti-anxiety drugs (such as benzodiazepines), antidepressants, and beta-blockers.

Anti-Anxiety Medications

Anti-anxiety medications can help reduce the symptoms of anxiety, panic attacks, or extreme fear and worry. The most common anti-anxiety medications are called benzodiazepines. Although benzodiazepines are sometimes used as first-line treatments for generalized anxiety disorder, they have both benefits and drawbacks.

Some benefits of benzodiazepines are that they are effective in relieving anxiety and take effect more quickly than antidepressant medications often prescribed for anxiety. Some drawbacks of benzodiazepines are that people can build up a tolerance to them if they are taken over a long period of time and they may need higher and higher doses to get the same effect. Some people may even become dependent on them.

To avoid these problems, doctors usually prescribe benzodiazepines for short periods of time, a practice that is especially helpful for older adults, people who have substance abuse problems, and people who become dependent on medication easily.

If people suddenly stop taking benzodiazepines,

they may have withdrawal symptoms, or their anxiety may return. Therefore, benzodiazepines should be tapered off slowly. When you and your doctor have decided it is time to stop the medication, the doctor will help you slowly and safely decrease your dose.

For long-term use, benzodiazepines are often considered a second-line treatment for anxiety (with antidepressants being considered a first-line treatment) as well as an "as-needed" treatment for any distressing flare-ups of symptoms.

A different type of anti-anxiety medication is *buspirone*. Buspirone is a non-benzodiazepine medication specifically indicated for the treatment of chronic anxiety, although it does not help everyone.

Antidepressants

Antidepressants are used to treat depression, but they can also be helpful for treating anxiety disorders. They may help improve the way your brain uses certain chemicals that control mood or stress. You may need to try several different antidepressant medicines before finding the one that improves your symptoms and has manageable side effects. A medication that has helped you or a close family member in the past will often be considered.

Antidepressants can take time to work, so it's important to give the medication a chance before reaching a conclusion about its effectiveness. If you begin taking antidepressants, do not stop taking them without the help of a doctor. When you and your doctor have decided it is time to stop the medication, the doctor will help you slowly and safely decrease your dose. Stopping them abruptly can cause withdrawal symptoms.

Antidepressants called selective serotonin reuptake inhibitors (SSRIs) and serotonin-norepinephrine reuptake inhibitors (SNRIs) are commonly used as first-line treatments for anxiety. Less-commonly used — but effective — treatments for anxiety disorders are older classes of antidepressants, such as tricyclic antidepressants and monoamine oxidase inhibitors (MAOIs).

Please Note: In some cases, children, teenagers, and young adults under 25 may experience an increase in suicidal thoughts or behavior when taking antidepressant medications, especially in the first few weeks after starting or when the dose is changed. Because of this, patients of all ages taking antidepressants should be watched closely, especially during the first few weeks of treatment.

Beta-Blockers

Although beta-blockers are most often used to treat high blood pressure, they can also be used to help relieve the physical symptoms of anxiety, such as rapid heartbeat, shaking, trembling, and blushing. These medications, when taken for a short period of time, can help people keep physical symptoms under control. They can also be used "as needed" to reduce acute anxiety, including as a preventive intervention for some predictable forms of performance anxieties.

Choosing the Right Medication

Some types of drugs may work better for specific types of anxiety disorders, so people should work closely with their doctor to identify which medication is best for them. Certain substances such as caffeine, some over-the-counter cold medicines, illicit drugs, and herbal supplements may aggravate the symptoms of anxiety disorders or interact with prescribed medication. Patients should talk with their doctor, so they can learn which substances are safe and which to avoid.

Choosing the right medication, medication dose, and treatment plan should be done under an expert's care and should be based on a person's needs and their medical situation. Your doctor may try several medicines before finding the right one.

You and your doctor should discuss:

- How well medications are working or might work to improve your symptoms
- Benefits and side effects of each medication
- Risk for serious side effects based on your medical history
- The likelihood of the medications requiring lifestyle changes
- Costs of each medication
- Other alternative therapies, medications, vitamins, and supplements you are taking and how these may affect your treatment; a combination of medication and psychotherapy is the best approach for many people with anxiety disorders
- How the medication should be stopped (Some drugs can't be stopped abruptly and must be tapered off slowly under a doctor's supervision).

Support Groups

Some people with anxiety disorders might benefit from joining a self-help or support group and sharing their problems and achievements with others. Internet chat rooms might also be useful, but any advice received over the internet should be used with caution, as Internet acquaintances have usually never seen each other and what has helped one person is not necessarily what is best for another. You should always check with your doctor before following any treatment advice found on the internet. Talking with a trusted friend or member of the clergy can also provide support, but it is not necessarily a sufficient alternative to care from a doctor or other health professional.

Stress Management Techniques

Stress management techniques and meditation can help people with anxiety disorders calm themselves and may enhance the effects of therapy. Research suggests that aerobic exercise can help some people manage their anxiety; however, exercise should not take the place of standard care and more research is needed.

Appendix A: Guide to Better Living

Note: Always consult your physician before making any changes to your diet, physical activity or life style.

Is your health condition requires that you make changes to your diet, physical activity, or life style? Are you thinking about being more active? Have you been trying to cut back on less healthy foods? Are you starting to eat better and move more but having a hard time sticking with these changes?

Old habits die hard. Changing your habits is a process that involves several stages. Sometimes it takes a while before changes become new habits. And, you may face roadblocks along the way.

Adopting new, healthier habits may protect you from serious health problems. New habits, like healthy eating and regular physical activity, may also help you manage your weight and have more energy. After a while, if you stick with these changes, they may become part of your daily routine.

The information below outlines four stages you may go through when changing your health habits or behavior. You will also find tips to help you improve your eating, physical activity habits, and overall health. The four stages of changing a health behavior are

- contemplation
- preparation
- action
- maintenance

What stage of change are you in?

Contemplation: "I'm thinking about it."

In this first stage, you are thinking about change and becoming motivated to get started.

You might be in this stage if you

- have been considering change but are not quite ready to start
- believe that your health, energy level, or overall well-being will improve if you develop new habits
- are not sure how you will overcome the roadblocks that may keep you from starting to change

Preparation: "I have made up my mind to take action."

In this next stage, you are making plans and thinking of specific ideas that will work for you.

You might be in this stage if you

- have decided that you are going to change and are ready to take action
- have set some specific goals that you would like to meet
- are getting ready to put your plan into action

Action: "I have started to make changes."

In this third stage, you are acting on your plan and making the changes you set out to achieve.

You might be in this stage if you

- have been making eating, physical activity, and other behavior changes in the last 6 months or so
- are adjusting to how it feels to eat healthier, be more active, and make other changes such as getting more sleep or reducing screen time
- have been trying to overcome things that sometimes block your success

Maintenance: "I have a new routine."

In this final stage, you have become used to your changes and have kept them up for more than 6 months.

You might be in this stage if

- your changes have become a normal part of your routine
- you have found creative ways to stick with your routine
- you have had slip-ups and setbacks but have been able to get past them and make progress

Did you find your stage of change? Read on for ideas about what you can do next.

Contemplation: Are you thinking of making changes?

Making the leap from thinking about change to taking action can be hard and may take time. Asking yourself about the pros (benefits) and cons (things that get in the way) of changing your habits may be helpful. How would life be better if you made some changes?

Think about how the benefits of healthy eating or regular physical activity might relate to your overall health. For example, suppose your blood glucose, also called blood sugar, is a bit high and you have a parent, brother, or sister who has type 2 diabetes. This means you also may develop type 2 diabetes. You may find that it is easier to be physically active and eat healthy knowing that it may help control blood glucose and protect you from a serious disease.

You may learn more about the benefits of changing your eating and physical activity habits from a health care professional. This knowledge may help you take action.

Look at the lists of pros and cons below. Find the items you believe are true for you. Think about factors that are important to you.

Healthy Eating

Pros

- have more energy
- improve my health
- lower my risk for health problems
- maintain a healthy weight
- feel proud of myself
- set an example for friends and family

Cons

- may spend more money and time on food
- may need to cook more often at home
- may need to eat less of foods I love
- may need to buy different foods
- may need to convince my family that we all have to eat healthier foods

Physical Activity

Pros	**Cons**
• improve my health	• takes too much time and energy
• reduce my risk for serious health problems	• it is too hot or cold outside
• feel better about myself	• feel self-conscious
• become stronger	• am nervous about my health
• have fun	• could hurt myself
• take time to care for myself	• am not good at being active
• meet new people and spend time with them	• do not know what to do
• have more energy	• have no one to be active with
• maintain a healthy weight	• am not young or fit enough
• become a role model for others	• keeps me from family and friends

Preparation: Have you made up your mind?

If you are in the preparation stage, you are about to take action. To get started, look at your list of pros and cons. How can you make a plan and act on it?

The chart below lists common roadblocks you may face and possible solutions to overcome roadblocks as you begin to change your habits. Think about these things as you make your plan.

Roadblock: I don't have time.

Solution: Make your new healthy habit a priority. Fit in physical activity whenever and wherever you can. Try taking the stairs or getting off the bus a stop early if it is safe to do so. Set aside one grocery shopping day a week, and make healthy meals that you can freeze and eat later when you don't have time to cook.

Roadblock: Healthy habits cost too much.

Solution: You can walk around the mall, a school track, or a local park for free. Eat healthy on a budget by buying in bulk and when items are on sale, and by choosing frozen or canned fruits and vegetables.

Roadblock: I can't make this change alone.

Solution: Recruit others to be active with you, which will help you stay motivated and safe. Consider signing up for a fun fitness class like salsa dancing. Get your family or coworkers on the healthy eating bandwagon. Plan healthy meals together with your family, or start a healthy potluck once a week at work.

Roadblock: I don't like physical activity.

Solution: Forget the old notion that being physically active means lifting weights in a gym. You can be active in many ways, including dancing, walking, or gardening. Make your own list of options that appeal to you. Explore options you never thought about, and stick with what you enjoy.

Roadblock: I don't like healthy foods.

Solution: Try making your old favorite recipes in healthier new ways. For example, you can trim fat from meats and reduce the amount of butter, sugar, and salt you cook with. Use low-fat cheeses or milk rather than whole-milk foods. Add a cup or two of broccoli, carrots, or spinach to casseroles or pasta.

Once you have made up your mind to change your habits, make a plan and set goals for taking action. Here are some ideas for making your plan:

- learn more about healthy eating (https://www.myplate.gov/)
- learn more about being active (see appendix B)
- make lists of
  - healthy foods that you like or may need to eat more of—or more often
  - foods you love that you may need to eat less often
  - things you could do to be more physically active
  - fun activities you like and could do more often, such as dancing

After making your plan, start setting goals for putting your plan into action. Start with small changes. For example, "I'm going to walk for 10 minutes, three times a week." What is the one step you can take right away?

Action: Have you started to make changes?

You are making real changes to your lifestyle, which is fantastic! To stick with your new habits

- review your plan
- look at the goals you set and how well you are meeting them
- overcome roadblocks by planning ahead for setbacks
- reward yourself for your hard work

Track your progress

- Tracking your progress helps you spot your strengths, find areas where you can improve, and stay on course. Record not only what you did, but how you felt while doing it—your feelings can play a role in making your new habits stick.
- Recording your progress may help you stay focused and catch setbacks in meeting your goals. Remember that a setback does not mean you have failed. All of us experience setbacks. The key is to get back on track as soon as you can.
- You can track your progress with online tools such as the NIH Body Weight Planner (https://www.youtube.com/watch?v=v1gluQwi eog). The NIH Body Weight Planner lets you tailor your calorie and physical activity plans to reach your personal goals within a specific time period.

Overcome roadblocks

- Remind yourself why you want to be healthier. Perhaps you want the energy to play with your nieces and nephews or to be able to carry your own grocery bags. Recall your reasons for making changes when slip-ups occur. Decide to take the first step to get back on track.

- Problem-solve to "outsmart" roadblocks. For example, plan to walk indoors, such as at a mall, on days when bad weather keeps you from walking outside.
- Ask a friend or family member for help when you need it, and always try to plan ahead. For example, if you know that you will not have time to be physically active after work, go walking with a coworker at lunch or start your day with an exercise video.

Reward yourself

- After reaching a goal or milestone, allow for a nonfood reward such as new workout gear or a new workout device. Also consider posting a message on social media to share your success with friends and family.
- Choose rewards carefully. Although you should be proud of your progress, keep in mind that a high-calorie treat or a day off from your activity routine are not the best rewards to keep you healthy.
- Pat yourself on the back. When negative thoughts creep in, remind yourself how much good you are doing for your health by moving more and eating healthier.

Maintenance: Have you created a new routine?

Make your future a healthy one. Remember that eating healthy, getting regular physical activity, and other healthy habits are lifelong behaviors, not one-time events. Always keep an eye on your efforts and seek ways to deal with the planned and unplanned changes in life.

Now that healthy eating and regular physical activity are part of your routine, keep things interesting, avoid slip-ups, and find ways to cope with what life throws at you.

Add variety and stay motivated

Mix up your routine with new physical activities and goals, physical activity buddies, foods, recipes, and rewards.

Deal with unexpected setbacks

Plan ahead to avoid setbacks. For example, find other ways to be active in case of bad weather, injury, or other issues that arise. Think of ways to eat healthy when traveling or dining out, like packing healthy snacks while on the road or sharing an entrée with a friend in a restaurant.

If you do have a setback, don't give up. Setbacks happen to everyone. Regroup and focus on meeting your goals again as soon as you can.

Challenge yourself!

Revisit your goals and think of ways to expand them. For example, if you are comfortable walking 5 days a week, consider adding strength training twice a week. If you have limited your saturated fat intake by eating less fried foods, try cutting back on added sugars, too. Small changes can lead to healthy habits worth keeping.

**When The Going Gets Tough,
Put One Foot in Front of The
Other and Just Keep Going.
Don't Give Up!**

Appendix B: How to Stay Active

Note: Always consult your physician before making any changes to your diet, physical activity or life style.

Physical activity may seem hard if you're overweight. You may get short of breath or tired quickly. Finding or affording the right clothes and equipment may be frustrating. Or, perhaps you may not feel comfortable working out in front of others.

The good news is you can overcome these challenges. Not only can you be active at any size, you can have fun and feel good at the same time.

Can anyone be active?

Research strongly shows that physical activity is safe for almost everyone. The health benefits of physical activity far outweigh the risks.

The activities discussed here are safe for most people. If you have problems moving or staying steady on your feet, or if you get out of breath easily, talk with a health care professional before you start. You also should talk with a health care professional if you are unsure of your health, have any concerns that physical activity may be unsafe for you, or have

- a chronic disease such as diabetes, high blood pressure, or heart disease
- a bone or joint problem—for example, in your back, knee, or hip—that could get worse if you change your physical activity level

Why should I be active?

Being active may help you live longer and protect you from developing serious health problems, such as type 2 diabetes, heart disease, stroke, and certain types of cancer. Regular physical activity is linked to many health benefits, such as

- lower blood pressure and blood glucose, or blood sugar
- healthy bones, muscles, and joints
- a strong heart and lungs
- better sleep at night and improved mood

The Physical Activity Guidelines for Americans define regular physical activity as at least 150 minutes a week of moderate-intensity aerobic activity, such as brisk walking. Brisk walking is a pace of 3 miles per hour or faster. A moderate-intensity activity makes you breathe harder but does not overwork or overheat you. You should also do muscle-strengthening activities at least 2 days a week.

You may reach this goal by starting with 5 minutes

of physical activity several times a day, 5 to 6 days a week. You could then gradually work up to 10 minutes per session, 3 times a day. If you do even more activity, you may gain even more health benefits.

When combined with healthy eating, regular physical activity may also help you control your weight. However, research shows that even if you can't lose weight or maintain your weight loss, you still can enjoy important health benefits from regular physical activity.

Physical activity also can be a lot of fun if you do activities you enjoy and are active with other people. Being active with others may give you a chance to meet new people or spend more time with family and friends. You also may inspire and motivate one another to get and stay active.

What do I need to know about becoming active?

Choosing physical activities that match your fitness level and health goals can help you stay motivated and keep you from getting hurt. You may feel some minor discomfort or muscle soreness when you first become active. These feelings should go away as you get used to your activity. However, if you feel sick to your stomach or have pain, you may have done too much. Go easier and then slowly build up your activity level. Some activities, such as walking or swimming, are less likely to cause injuries.

If you have been inactive, start slowly and see how you feel. Gradually increase how long and how often you are active. If you need guidance, check with a health care or certified fitness professional.

Here are some tips for staying safe during physical activity:

- Wear the proper safety gear, such as a bike helmet if you are bicycling.
- Make sure any sports equipment you use works and fits properly.
- Look for safe places to be active. For instance, walk in well-lit areas where other people are around. Be active with a friend or group.
- Stay hydrated to replace the body fluids you lose through sweating and to prevent you from getting overheated.
- If you are active outdoors, protect yourself from the sun with sunscreen and a hat or protective visor and clothing.
- Wear enough clothing to keep warm in cold or windy weather. Layers are best.

If you don't feel right, stop your activity. If you have any of the following warning signs, stop and seek help right away:

- pain, tightness, or pressure in your chest or neck, shoulder, or arm
- extreme shortness of breath
- dizziness or sickness

Check with a health care professional about what to do if you have any of these warning signs. If your activity is causing pain in your joints, feet, ankles, or legs, you also should consult a health care professional to see if you may need to change the type or amount of activity you are doing.

What kinds of activities can I do?

You don't need to be an athlete or have special skills or equipment to make physical activity part of your life. Many types of activities you do every day, such as walking your dog or going up and down steps at home or at work, may help improve your health.

Try different activities you enjoy. If you like an activity, you're more likely to stick with it. Anything that gets you moving around, even for a few minutes at a time, is a healthy start to getting fit.

Walking

Walking is free and easy to do—and you can do it

almost anywhere. Walking will help you

- burn calories
- improve your fitness
- lift your mood
- strengthen your bones and muscles

If you are concerned about safety, try walking in a shopping mall or park where it is well lit and other people are around. Many malls and parks have benches where you can take a quick break. Walking with a friend or family member is safer than walking alone and may provide the social support you need to meet your activity goals.

If you don't have time for a long walk, take several short walks instead. For example, instead of a 30-minute walk, add three 10-minute walks to your day. Shorter spurts of activity are easier to fit into a busy schedule.

Walking tips

- Wear comfortable, well-fitting walking shoes with a lot of support, and socks that absorb sweat.
- Dress for the weather if you are walking outdoors. In cold weather, wear layers of clothing you can remove if you start getting too warm. In hot weather, protect yourself against the sun and heat.

- Warm up by walking more slowly for the first few minutes. Cool down by slowing your pace.

Dancing

Dancing can be a lot of fun while it tones your muscles, strengthens your heart and lungs, and boosts your mood. You can dance at a health club, dance studio, or even at home. Just turn on some lively music and start moving. You also can dance to a video on your TV or computer.

If you have trouble standing on your feet for a long time, try dancing while sitting down. Chair dancing lets you move your arms and legs to music while taking the weight off your feet.

Bicycling

Riding a bicycle spreads your weight among your arms, back, and hips. For outdoor biking, you may want to try a mountain bike. Mountain bikes have wider tires and are sturdier than bikes with thinner tires. You can buy a larger seat to make biking more comfortable.

For indoor biking, you may want to try a recumbent bike. On this type of bike, you sit lower to the ground with your legs reaching forward to the pedals. Your body is in more of a reclining position, which may feel better than sitting straight up. The seat on a recumbent bike is also wider than the seat on a regular bike.

If you decide to buy a bike, check how much weight it can support to make sure it is safe for you.

Workout clothing tips

- Clothes made of fabrics that absorb sweat are best for working out.
- Comfortable, lightweight clothes allow you to move more easily.
- Tights or spandex shorts are the best bottoms to wear to prevent inner-thigh chafing.
- Women should wear a bra that provides extra support during physical activity.

Water workouts

Swimming and water workouts put less stress on your joints than walking, dancing, or biking. If your feet, back, or joints hurt when you stand, water activities may be best for you. If you feel self-conscious about wearing a bathing suit, you can wear shorts and a T-shirt while you swim.

Exercising in water

- Lets you be more flexible. You can move your body in water in ways you may not be able to on land.

- Reduces your risk of hurting yourself. Water provides a natural cushion, which keeps you from pounding or jarring your joints.
- Helps prevent sore muscles.
- Keeps you cool, even when you are working hard.

You don't need to know how to swim to work out in water. You can do shallow- or deep-water exercises at either end of the pool without swimming. For instance, you can do laps while holding onto a kickboard and kicking your feet. You also can walk or jog across the width of the pool while moving your arms.

For shallow-water workouts, the water level should be between your waist and chest. During deep-water workouts, most of your body is underwater. For safety and comfort, wear a foam belt or life jacket.

Tips for protecting your hair

If you're worried that pool water will damage or mess up your hair, try these tips:

- Use a swim cap to help protect your hair from pool chemicals and getting wet.
- Wear a natural hairstyle, short braids, locs, or twists, which may be easier to style after a water workout.

- Buy a shampoo to remove chlorine buildup, available at most drug stores, if your hair feels dry or damaged after a pool workout.

Strength training

Strength training involves using free weights, weightlifting machines, resistance bands, or your own body weight to make your muscles stronger. Lower-body strength training will improve your balance and prevent falls.

Strength training may help you

- build and maintain strong muscles as you get older
- continue to perform activities of daily living, such as carrying groceries or moving furniture
- keep your bones strong, which may help prevent osteoporosis and fractures

If you are just starting out, using a weightlifting machine may be safer than dumbbells. As you get fit, you may want to add free-weight exercises with dumbbells.

You do not need a weight bench or large dumbbells to do strength training at home. You can use a pair of hand weights to do bicep curls. You can also use your own body weight: for example, get up and down from a chair.

Proper form is very important when lifting weights. You may hurt yourself if you don't lift weights properly. You may want to schedule a session with a certified fitness professional to learn which exercises to do and how to do them safely. Check with your health insurer about whether your health plan covers these services.

If you decide to buy a home gym, check how much weight it can support to make sure it is safe for you.

Strength-training tips

- Aim for at least 2 days per week of strengthen-training activities.
- Try to perform each exercise 8 to 12 times. If that's too hard, the weight you are lifting is too heavy. If it's too easy, your weight is too light.
- Try to exercise all the major muscle groups. These groups include the muscles of the legs, hips, chest, back, abdomen, shoulders, and arms.
- Don't work the same muscles 2 days in a row. Your muscles need time to recover.

Mind and body exercise

Your local hospital or fitness, recreation, or community center may offer classes such as yoga, tai chi, or Pilates. You also may find some of these workouts online and can download them to a computer, smart phone, or other device. These types of activities may help you

- become stronger and more flexible
- feel more relaxed
- improve balance and posture

Your local hospital or fitness, recreation, or community center may offer classes such as yoga, tai chi, or Pilates.

These classes also can be a lot of fun and add variety to your workout routine. If some movements are hard to do or you have injuries you are concerned about, talk with the instructor about how to adapt the exercises and poses to meet your needs—or start with a beginner's class.

Daily life activities

Daily life activities, such as cleaning out the attic or washing the car, are great ways to get moving. Small changes can add more physical activity to your day and improve your health. Try these:

- Take 2- to 3-minute walking breaks at work several times a day, if possible.
- Stand, walk, or stretch in place during TV commercials.
- Take the stairs instead of the elevator or escalator whenever you can.

- Park farther from where you are going and walk the rest of the way.

Even a shopping trip can be exercise because it provides a chance to walk and carry your bags. Chores such as mowing the lawn, raking leaves, and gardening also count.

Where can I be active?

You can find many fun places to be active. Having more than one place may keep you from getting bored. Here are some options:

- Join or take a class at a local fitness, recreation, or community center.
- Enjoy the outdoors by taking a hike or going for a walk in a safe local park, neighborhood, or mall.
- Work out in the comfort of your own home with a workout video or by finding a fitness channel on your TV, tablet, or other mobile device.

Tips for choosing a fitness center

- Make sure the center has exercise equipment for people who weigh more and staff to show you how to use it.
- Ask if the center has any special classes for people just starting out, older adults, or people with mobility or health issues.

- See if you can try out the center or take a class before you join.
- Try to find a center close to work or home. The quicker and easier the center is to get to, the better your chances of using it often.
- Make sure you understand the rules for joining and ending your membership, what your membership fee covers, any related costs, and the days and hours of operation.

How can I get past my roadblocks?

You most likely will face roadblocks that keep you from meeting your physical activity goals. Think about what keeps you from being active, then try to come up with creative ways to address those roadblocks. Here are a few examples to help you get started:

Barrier: I don't have enough time.

Solution: Instead of doing one long workout session, build in three 10-minute bursts of activity during your day, such as a brisk walk. Even standing up instead of sitting at your desk has benefits.

Barrier: I just don't like exercise.

Solution: Good news! You don't have to run a marathon or go to the gym all the time to benefit from being active. To make physical activity more fun, try something you enjoy doing, such as dancing to the radio or taking a yoga class with friends. Many people find they start to like exercise better the more they do it.

Barrier: I'm worried about my health or getting hurt.

Solution: If you have a hard time being active because of your health, talk with a health care professional first. A certified fitness professional can also guide you on how to be active safely.

Barrier: I feel self-conscious working out in front of others.

Solution: Start being active at home until you feel more confident. Be active with friends who will support and encourage you.

How can I stick with my physical activity plan?

Sticking with a plan to be physically active can be a challenge. Online tools such as the NIH Body Weight Planner (https://www.youtube.com/watch?v=v1gluQwieog) can help. The NIH Body Weight Planner lets you tailor your calorie and physical activity plans to reach your personal goals within a specific time period.

You also can download fitness apps that let you enter information to track your progress using a computer or smart phone or other mobile device.

Devices you can wear, such as pedometers and fitness trackers, may help you count steps, calories, and minutes of physical activity. Trackers can help you set goals and monitor progress. You wear most of these devices on your wrist like a watch, or clipped to your clothing.

Keeping an activity journal is another good way to help you stay motivated and on track to reach your fitness goals.

Set goals. As you track your activity, try to set specific short- and long-term goals. For example, instead of "I will be more active," set a goal such as "I will take a walk after lunch at least 2 days a week." Getting started with a doable goal is a good way to form a new habit. A short-term goal may be to walk 5 to 10 minutes, 5 days a week. A long-term goal may be to do at least 150 minutes of moderate-intensity physical activity a week.

Get support. Ask a family member or friend to be active with you. Your workout buddy can help make your activities more fun and can cheer you on and help you meet your goals.

Track progress. You may not feel as though you

are making progress, but when you look back at where you started, you may be pleasantly surprised. Making regular activity part of your life is a big step. Start slowly and praise yourself for every goal you set and achieve.

Review your goals. Did you meet your goals? If not, why? Are they doable? Did you hit a roadblock trying to meet your goal? What will you do differently next week? Brainstorm some options to overcome future roadblocks. Ask a friend or family member to help support your goals.

Pick nonfood rewards. Whether your goal is to be active 15 minutes a day, to walk farther than you did last week, or simply to stay positive, recognizing your efforts is an important part of staying on track. Decide how you will reward yourself. Some ideas for rewards include getting new music to charge you up or buying new workout gear.

Be patient with yourself. Don't get discouraged if you have setbacks from time to time. If you can't achieve your goal the first time or can only stick to your goals for part of the week, remind yourself that this is all part of establishing new habits.

Look ahead. Try to focus on what you will do differently moving forward, rather than on what went wrong. Pat yourself on the back for trying.

Most importantly, don't give up. Any movement, even for a short time, is a good thing. Each activity you add to your life is another step toward a healthier you.